BREAST CANCER TREATMENT:

A Guide for You and your Loved Ones

By

Dr. DENNIS J. THOMAS

Table of contents

Introduction

How is breast cancer treated?

Breast cancer is treated in different ways than one. The treatment depends on the kind of breast cancer and how far it has spread to the other part of the body. Individuals with breast cancer usually get more than one kind of treatment. Breast cancer treatments are Chemotherapy, hormonal therapy, immunotherapy, radiation therapy, targeted therapy, and surgery. Different Specialists usually cooperate to treat breast cancer.

Doctors that perform operations are Surgeons. Doctors who treat cancer with medicine are Medical oncologists. Doctors who treat cancer with radiation are Radiation oncologists.

Chapter 1

CHEMOTHERAPY

Chemotherapy is a drug that fights and kills cancer cells or slows their division and development. Chemotherapy drugs may be given in pill form or by infusion or injection and are often used with other treatments: radiation therapy, targeted therapy, and surgery.

When given through injection, chemotherapy treatment is passed into a vein with a needle rapidly, requiring only a few minutes. If it is an infusion, it does require a few hours. In some cases, there can be a need to have a central venous catheter, for example, a PICC line or port introduced to give a steady infusion site. Whether you are to take an injection or infusion, chemotherapy is what that can be done at your doctor's office, or in a hospital.

Types of chemotherapy

Even though it is not every cancer patient that needs chemotherapy, there are many cases when it may be used.

After surgery: When chemotherapy is required after breast cancer surgery, it's called adjuvant breast cancer chemotherapy. This type of chemotherapy is to eliminate any leftover cancer cells that might not have been eliminated during surgery and or radiation therapy. This also is to prevent this cancer from spreading to different parts of the body and to minimize the risk of recurrence.

Before surgery: Chemotherapy may be administered before breast cancer surgery this is called neoadjuvant breast cancer chemotherapy. This type of chemotherapy usually makes breast-conserving surgery easy and possible by assisting with diminishing the size of large breast tumors and eliminating cancer cells. It likewise helps cancer specialists decide the impact a specific routine is having on the breast tumor.

Treatment for advanced breast cancer: In patients whose breast cancer has spread (metastasized) past the breast and close by regions, chemotherapy may be the first treatment used. The number of times to receive chemotherapy treatment is determined by your particular situation (cancer type and stage), which also include how well the chemotherapy treatment is working and whether you can withstand the treatment.

The type of chemotherapy drug taken, and when it is taken in conjunction with other types of therapies, relies upon the patient, the type of breast cancer, and its stage.

Side effects of chemotherapy

Chemotherapy drugs do attack fast-developing cells all through the body, including cancer cells. Some normal cells in the body also do develop rapidly and may be attacked by chemotherapy drugs. Those cells include:

- Immune cells and those tracked down in bone marrow
- Cells in the digestive system
- Hair follicle cells

When chemotherapy attacks these normal cells, it may cause short-term side effects on the patient, but generally disappear after treatment, for example:

- Weight loss
- Hair loss
- Constipation

- Fatigue
- High risk of infection
- Nausea and diarrhea
- Loss of appetite

There are also long-term side effects from chemotherapy. In women who haven't started menopause, chemotherapy may Causes are:

- Infertility
- Premature menopause

These side effects are more probable the older you are at the beginning of treatment, and if they do happen, you might encounter a more serious risk of bone loss and/or osteoporosis.

It's essential to take note that getting pregnant during chemotherapy increases the risk of birth defects, so make sure you ask your doctor about suitable contraceptive medication during treatment.

Uncommon long-term side effects of some chemotherapy drugs include:

- Heart damage
- Nerve damage

- Chemo brain (in which memory is decreased, a side effect that lasts for several years).

Furthermore, once in a while, chemotherapy medications may increase your chance of getting leukemia, it is common 10 years after treatment.

Side effects of chemotherapy depend on the patient, the drug(s) taken, and the dosage taken. At Cancer Treatment Centers of America® (CTCA), your health provider team will be pretty much proactive to help combat the side effects, so you can allow your chemotherapy treatment. Your health provider team may likewise offer different supportive services based on your needs, to help manage side effects. A good diet, naturopathic support, and mind-body medication may reduce chemotherapy-related side effects so you can keep on taking part in the exercises you appreciate.

Chapter 2
RADIATION THERAPY

Radiation therapy is the use of high-energy X-rays or other types of radiation to kill cancer cells. Breast cancer patients may get/need one or a combination of radiation therapies that are grouped into two fundamental categories:

- External beam radiation therapy
- Accelerated partial breast irradiation

Radiation therapy is regularly suggested for breast cancer patients after a breast lump or a tumor has been taken out, to kill any remaining cancer cells that may have been left behind. Radiation therapy can also be used with other types of therapies, like chemotherapy or hormone therapy. The length of radiation treatment therapy depends on different variables, including the type of therapy used and the stage of breast cancer.

External beam radiation therapy (EBRT)

The most widely recognized type of radiation therapy for breast cancer, EBRT is administered after other treatments are completed.

In EBRT, a collection of rays of radiation, a high-energy X-ray, is centered on the spot where the cancer was taken out. If a lumpectomy was done, the patient may need to receive EBRT to the whole breast, a procedure called whole-breast radiation. EBRT may likewise be extended to nearby lymph nodes. A few benefits of EBRT for breast cancer patients include:

- It is quick, painless, and performed as an outpatient procedure.
- EBRT is targeted to the treatment region, unlike chemotherapy which circulates throughout the body.
- No patient during radiation therapy is radioactive, and there's no risk of radioactivity to your loved ones.

Types of EBRT

Intensity-modulated radiation therapy (IMRT):
High-level software is used to administer an exact dose of radiation to the region where a tumor was removed. A computer-controlled gadget called a linear accelerator passed radiation in sculptured doses that match the three-dimensional shape of the target.

Advantages of IMRT for breast cancer

- IMRT uses a high-level computer program to plan your radiation dosage in three dimensions.
- IMRT sends radiation to the target region and regulates the intensity of the radiation beams, assisting with saving healthy tissue.

IMRT breast cancer radiation therapy can be used with some other treatments. It is a suitable option for those who have previously had breast cancer radiation treatment and are encountering recurrent tumors in the treated region.

Image-guided radiation therapy (IGRT)

IGRT utilizes images during radiation therapy. Images are taken before and during treatment, and images taken during treatment are compared to images taken before treatment starts. This assists doctors with positioning the radiation as accurately as possible.

Stereotactic radiation therapy (SRT)

This treatment conveys a large and exact dose to a small cancer region. The patient must be still. A head frame or individual body molds assist limit movement. SRT is much of the time given as a single treatment or in less than 10 treatments. Certain individuals might require more than one course of SRT.

Proton beam therapy

This treatment utilizes protons as opposed to x-rays. At high energy, protons can eliminate cancer cells. The protons go to the designated cancer/tumor and drop a particular dose of radiation therapy. Not at all like x-ray beams, very little radiation dose goes past the tumor with proton treatment. This limits harm to nearby tissue.

Three-dimensional conformal radiation (3D-CRT)

During this type of radiation treatment, detailed 3-dimensional images of the cancer are gotten from computed tomography (CT) or magnetic resonance imaging (MRI) scans. The treatment team utilizes these images to aim the radiation beam at the cancer region. With this procedure, the treatment team can securely use higher doses of radiation therapy and reduce harm to healthy tissues. This brings down the risk of side effects.

Accelerated partial breast irradiation (APBI):

This is a breast radiation therapy that delivers focused radiation specifically to the part of the breast where the cancer cell was removed from.

Advantages of APBI for breast cancer

- Radiation is directed specifically to the tumor cavity.
- Since the radiation is targeted to the affected part, it attacks less healthy tissue and organs near the

breasts, which include the lungs, heart, ribs, muscles, and skin.

- It can be delivered within a short schedule than some other types of radiation therapies for breast cancer.

Types of APBI

High-dose-rate (HDR) brachytherapy: This is a type of radiation therapy that is internal, which delivers radiation from the placed implants close to or inside the tumor(s) in the patient body.

Advantages of HDR brachytherapy include:

- It delivers the needed and concentrated dose of radiation directly to the region where the tumor was removed from.
- The radiation exposure to healthy surrounding breast tissue is limited, which reduces the side effects of radiation therapy.

- The catheters are removed after a series of treatments and no radioactive materials are left to stay in the body again.

AccuBoost®: This is a breast-conservation therapy that delivers the targeted dose of radiation straight to the tissue surrounding the cancer tumor.

Advantages of AccuBoost are:

- The treatment may be done in an outpatient setting.
- The targeted dose is to help to send the radiation treatment to the lumpectomy site as much as it can.
- It helps to deliver a measured dose that matches the size, shape, and location of the target region. AccuBoost works to limit hazards to the breast.
- It is designed to limit radiation-related side effects.

Intraoperative radiation therapy (IORT):

- IORT is done immediately after the removal of the breast lump before the lumpectomy incision is closed. Doses of radiation are focused straight on the surgery site and it is sometimes the only radiation therapy most patients would have. In rare cases, additional EBRT therapy may be used.

- To be eligible for IORT, the patient must be eligible for surgery. This treatment is generally reserved for patients with an early stage of breast cancer.

Side effects of radiation therapy

Radiation therapy for breast cancer may bring some effects on the patient, either short-term or long-term side effects. Short-term side effects of radiation include:

- Redness or discoloration of the skin
- Fatigue
- Breast pain and/or swelling

Long-term side effects are:

- Bone weakness and fractures
- Nerve damage that may lead to weakness, numbness, or pain
- Damage to the lymph system resulting in lymphedema
- Damage to other organs exposed to radiation
- Difficulty breastfeeding.
- Changes to the feel or size of the breast

Chapter 3
TARGETED THERAPY

Targeted therapies are for the treatment of certain types of breast cancer. Specifically, they only focus on proteins that control or involve in how cancer grows, divides, and spreads in the patient body.

Targeted therapy is sometimes used with other cancer treatments like chemotherapy and radiation therapy because with time cancer cells may become resistant to targeted therapies.

When are targeted therapies used?

Targeted therapies have improved outcomes in some patients with hormone receptor-positive and HER2-positive cancers. HER2-positive breast cancer is the one that has the highest level of the HER2 protein on the surface of the breast cancer cells. This causes cancer cells to grow and spread faster.

Doctors do advise that women who have invasive breast cancer get HER2 test done using tissue from a biopsy or surgery with one of these two tests:

- Immunohistochemical stains (IHC)
- Fluorescent in situ hybridization (FISH)

Cancer can be hormone receptor-positive. Both normal breast cells and some breast cancer cells do have receptors. Estrogen and progesterone are hormones that can attach to receptors or proteins located in or on cells. This can also cause cancer to grow.

Hormone receptor-positive cancers usually grow slowly and may have better short-term outcomes. These types of cancers sometimes reoccur.

An immunohistochemistry test is used to determine whether cancer cells have these hormone receptors or not in or on them. A positive result means that at least one percent of the patient's cells have estrogen or progesterone receptors.

Targeted therapies might also be used to treat:

- Triple-positive cancers, which means estrogen receptor-positive, progesterone receptor-positive, and HER2-positive.

- Triple-negative cancers, which means estrogen receptor-negative, progesterone receptor-negative, and HER2-negative.
- Cancer patients that have a mutation in BRCA1 or BRCA2 genes.

When breast cancer is diagnosed early, targeted therapy treatments may help kill this cancer. When combined with chemotherapy, targeted therapy helps in lowering the risk of returning cancer.

Targeted therapy drugs for breast cancer type

HER2-positive breast cancers respond to drugs that target the protein. Some cancers are HER2-positive and ER- and PR-positive. Those would be treated with a mixture of drugs to target all those types of cancer.

HER2-positive cancer treatments include:

- Monoclonal antibodies
- Kinase inhibitor
- Antibody-drug conjugates

Monoclonal antibodies include trastuzumab, which:

- Is also known as Herceptin®, Ogivri®, Herzuma®, Ontruzant®, Trazimera™, Kanjinti™ and Herceptin Hylecta™.
- Is an intravenous (IV) drug or an injection.
- Can be used alone or in conjunction with chemotherapy for breast cancer.
- Is usually given for six months or a year, at three-week intervals,(sometimes longer).
- Can also be used to treat cancer that has spread to other parts of the body.

Another monoclonal antibody is pertuzumab (Perjeta®), which:

- Is an intravenous drug
- Can be given with trastuzumab and chemotherapy.

These treatments can be used in both early and advanced breast cancer.

A third monoclonal antibody option is margetuximab (Margenza™), which:

- Is an intravenous drug.
- Can be used with chemotherapy for advanced breast cancer.
- Is used for metastatic breast cancer after the other targeted therapies have been used.

Sometimes, some people need a mixture of these targeted therapies for the treatment of HER2-positive cancers. The U.S. Food and Drug Administration (FDA) approved the drug, Phesgo™, a mixture of two drugs: trastuzumab and pertuzumab, delivered in a subcutaneous form. The drug also includes an additional medicine, hyaluronidase, and its side effects may include nasal congestion and drainage.

For hormone receptor-positive cancers, various targeted treatment options exist.

Some drugs are to block what are known as CDKs (cyclin-dependent kinases). CDK4 and CDK6 inhibitors are to slow cancer growth in women with advanced hormone receptor-positive cancer. Some are given in combination with other drugs, depending on the patient's menstrual or menopausal status. They are in pill form.

Other treatment options include an mTOR inhibitor and a P13K inhibitor.

- mTOR inhibitor: Everolimus (Afinitor®) is used in many patients who are post-menopausal and have advanced cancer that is ER- or PR-positive.
  It also blocks a protein that helps cells grow and divide. It may increase the effectiveness of hormone therapy drugs.
- P13K inhibitor: Alpelisib (Piqray®) may help stop cancer cells from growing and is taken as a pill, once daily.

Women with BRCA1 or BRCA2 genetic mutation may consider targeted therapy that blocks the proteins and helps to keep cancerous cells intact.

PARP inhibitors also block PARP proteins and make tumor cells die. These drugs are in pill form and are taken twice daily. They are usually used by women who have metastasized cancer and who have already had chemotherapy.

Triple-negative breast cancer is when your cancer does not make HER2 protein and it doesn't have estrogen or progesterone receptors.

A monoclonal antibody targeted therapy used in this type of cancer is sacituzumab govitecan (Trodelvy®):

- It is an intravenous treatment.
- Is paired with chemotherapy and delivers chemotherapy medication to the cells.
- It can also be used as a lone treatment to treat metastasized cancer after two chemotherapy treatments.

Side effects

Targeted therapies may cause different side effects that range in severity and duration, depending on your treatment plan.

Some are mild, like rash and skin changes, while others may be more severe. Since the side effects vary on the type of targeted therapy taken, it's important to speak with your doctor about the side effects you should expect with your treatment plan, and what you can do to manage them throughout your regimen.

Chapter 4
IMMUNOTHERAPY

Immunotherapy is one of the types of treatment for cancer that triggers the body's immune system to attack and kill the cancer cells. Cancer cells do not die normally like normal cells. They rapidly grow, divide and spread.

These abnormal cells usually change, or mutate, helping them to attack the immune system, which protects the body from disease and infections. Cancer immunotherapy drugs are to alert the immune system about these mutated cells so it can find and destroy them.

The important function of the immune system is to differentiate normal cells in the body from foreign cells.

The immune system is always on alert to attack any foreign invaders, such as viruses, bacteria, or fungi. Lymph nodes make up most of the immune system. White blood cells, including lymphocytes such as "T cells," fight infection and cancer. When a foreign invader is detected, the entire immune system is alerted through chemical signals.

The immune system depends on receptor proteins in certain immune cells to detect invaders. At certain checkpoints, when activated or deactivated, these receptors allow it to distinguish between healthy and invading cells. The work of the checkpoints is to keep the immune system from attacking healthy and normal cells.

Cancer cells don't trigger an immune response because they are the body's cells that have mutated, so those once-healthy cells no longer behave like normal cells. Because the immune system doesn't recognize the differences between normal cells and cancer cells, these cancer cells can continue to grow, divide, and spread throughout the body.

How immunotherapy sparks the immune system to help fight cancer

Immunotherapies use different methods to attack tumor cells. Immunotherapy types fall into three general categories:

- Checkpoint inhibitors, where cancer cells trick the immune system by signaling to the immune system and thinking their healthy cells are disrupted, now exposing them to attack by the immune system.
- Cytokines, Protein molecules that help regulate and direct the immune system are synthesized in a laboratory and then injected into the body in larger doses than are produced naturally, this helps in attacking cancer cells.
- Cancer vaccines, may reduce the risk of cancer by attacking different viruses that cause cancer, or may treat cancer by stimulating the immune system to attack cancer cells in a specific part of the body.

Immunotherapy may be used as a lone treatment or with other cancer treatments, such as surgery, chemotherapy, radiation therapy, and targeted therapy.

Some of the drugs used in immunotherapy?

Checkpoint inhibitor drugs target the PD-1 and the CTLA-4 receptors. Common checkpoint inhibitors include:

- Ipilimumab (Yervoy®)
- Pembrolizumab (Keytruda®)
- Nivolumab (Opdivo®)
- Atezolizumab (Tecentriq®)

Common cytokines used in cancer therapy include:

- Interleukin-2 (IL-2)
- Interferons-alpha (IFN-alpha)

Tumor-agnostic therapies

The FDA approved immunotherapy to treat cancers with specific genetic features, regardless of where in the body they originate. These treatments called tumor-agnostic therapies may be used to treat these cancers:

- Solid tumors with microsatellite instability-high (MSI-h) or mismatch repair deficiency (dMMR): These tumors may have unstable strands of DNA or they are unable to repair DNA damage.

- Solid tumors with high tumor mutation burden (TMB-h): These tumors have cells with a high number of different gene mutations, which may make them more likely to respond to immunotherapy.

Immunotherapy side effect

Immunotherapy may cause different side effects—many are flu-like symptoms—which include:

- Nausea or vomiting
- Mouth sores
- Rashes or itching
- Diarrhea
- Fatigue
- High blood pressure
- Headaches
- Fluid buildup, usually in the legs
- Fever or chills
- Pain or weakness

The side effects of immunotherapy generally become less severe after the first treatment.

Throughout your treatment, your care team will provide integrative care services, including diet support, naturopathic support, pain management, oncology rehabilitation, behavioral health, and spiritual support. These therapies may help reduce side effects and improve your overall quality of life during immunotherapy.

Types of immunotherapy

The importance of immunotherapy is to reset the body's immune system to be able to find and attack cancer cells. The different types of immunotherapy work in different ways and have their risks and advantages. Your care team will recommend any of these treatments based on the type of cancer and stage you have.

Monoclonal or therapeutic antibodies are developed in a laboratory and injected into the body. Some mark cancerous cells so that the immune system can identify and kill them. Others stop the growth of cancer cells or cause self-destruction.

CAR T-cell therapy has many names which include: adoptive cell therapy, adoptive immunotherapy, and immune cell therapy. Essentially, your care team takes out white blood cells from your tumor and grows them in a laboratory, strengthens them, and increases their natural ability to fight cancer. These cells are grown in large batches and injected back into the body to fight cancer.

Immune checkpoint inhibitors are types of drug that removes natural blockades within the body, which keeps the immune system in check. Without the natural blockades, the immune system may overreact—like in autoimmune diseases. But cancers will often use these blockades, or proteins, to hide from the immune system. With these blockades removed through checkpoint inhibitors, the body can respond more strongly to the cancer cells.

Cancer vaccine, also called immunotherapeutic or treatment vaccines, helps to boost the immune system response when you have cancer already. They aren't preventative vaccines.

Cytokines are proteins that are created by your body during natural infections that play an important role in stimulating your immune system cells. By supplementing the body's natural cytokines, these help to boost immune cells and move them toward their target which is the tumor.

Immune system modulators also called immunomodulators: are drugs that boost the body's immune reaction. There are different immunomodulators and they act in different ways—some focus specifically on certain parts of the immune system, while others act across the whole body.

Immunotherapy may be given as an IV medication into the vein, pills as an oral medication, capsules, or topical medication on your skin.

Differences between immunotherapy and chemotherapy

Chemotherapy drugs are used to attack fast-developing cells throughout the body, immunotherapy triggers the immune system of the body to be able to identify and attack the cancer cells.

Chemotherapy can't differentiate between the cells, it affects both fast-growing cancerous cells and also normal fast-growing cells, like those responsible for hair, and skin growth. That's why side effects like hair loss, nausea and vomiting, and skin and nail changes are more common and sometimes more severe with chemotherapy.

Risks of immunotherapy

The risks of immunotherapy depend on the type of immunotherapy used, the type of cancer and stage, the patient's general health condition, and the current treatment regimen. Each treatment has its different side effects, and patients may respond differently to the same treatment.

In general, there are side effects when you make the immune system function on the "high side." When you get a vaccine, you may experience symptoms like—fever, chills, fatigue, weakness, nausea, muscle aches

, and headache—because the immune system is working. This treatment may also cause a skin rash.

Chapter 5

HORMONE THERAPY

Hormone therapy may be part of your treatments if you've been diagnosed with breast cancer.

Hormone therapy may likewise be referred to as hormonal or endocrine treatment, this cancer treatment is not the same as menopausal hormone replacement therapy (HRT), which refers to the use of supplemental chemicals to assist with relieving the symptoms of menopause.

Certain tumors depend on chemicals to develop. In these cases, chemical treatment might slow or stop their spread by impeding the body's capacity to create these specific chemicals or changing how chemical receptors act in the body.

Breast and prostate tumors are the types of cancer that are usually treated with hormone therapy. Most breast tumors have either estrogen -receptor (ER) or progesterone (PR) receptors, or both, and that implies they need these hormones to develop and spread. Hormone therapy assists with making these hormones less accessible to developing cancer cells.

Hormone therapy is accessible through pills, injections, or surgery that eliminates hormone-creating organs, specifically the ovaries in women. It's commonly suggested alongside other cancer therapies.

If hormone therapy is important for your treatment plan, examine likely dangers or aftereffects with your doctors, so you know what's in store and can do whatever it takes to lessen them. Tell the doctors pretty much the entirety of your different meds to stay away from connections.

Types of hormone therapy

Aromatase inhibitors

Aromatase inhibitors — for example, anastrozole (Arimidex®), letrozole (Femara®), and exemestane (Aromasin®) — work by deactivating aromatase, which the body uses to make estrogen in the ovaries and different tissues.

These meds are used basically for women who are in their menopause stage. Estrogen creation declines decisively after menopause. Women in their premenopausal stage produce a lot of aromatase for the inhibitors to work. (Aromatase inhibitor medications might be endorsed for youthful ladies if they're given medication to suppress ovarian capability.)

Ask your healthcare provider whether you may gain from aromatase inhibitors given your cancer details. Patients may get aromatase inhibitors before surgery, so that the tumors can get shrink for easy removal, or after other treatments to keep cancer from returning. These medications can also be used for breast cancer counteraction for specific individuals who are at high risk.

Side effects: Hot blazes, night sweats, vaginal dryness.

Selective estrogen receptor modulators (SERMs)

Selective estrogen receptor modulators (SERMs) — include tamoxifen (Nolvadex®), raloxifene (Evista®), and toremifene (Fareston®) — specifically block estrogen from specific tissues, in particular the breast, while expanding its accessibility in different regions like the bones.

An oncologist may suggest SERMs after surgery for early ER-positive breast cancer, to lessen the possibilities that it recurs. They can also be used to treat advanced

breast cancer and to also prevent breast cancer in those with high risk.

Side effects: blood clot, bone loss, mood swings, depression, loss of sex drive.

Fulvestrant (Faslodex)

Fulvestrant ties to estrogen receptors, totally preventing the hormone from joining the receptors.

It is used for women who have advanced ER-positive breast cancer that has spread after the treatment with other types of hormone therapy. It's also used for postmenopausal women with ER-positive, HER-negative cancers, who have not undergone other hormone therapy

Side effects: sickness, spewing, clogging, weakness, back torment, bone agony, joint agony, migraines, and breathing issues.

Ovarian suppression

Ovarian suppression slows the development of hormone receptor-positive breast cancer in premenopausal women.

Ovarian suppression deals with using drugs or surgery to keep the ovaries from making estrogen. This stops menstruation and brings down the hormone levels in the body, so cancer can't get the estrogen it needs to develop.

Side effects: bone loss, mood swings, depression, loss of sex interest, night sweats, vaginal dryness.

Chapter 6

BREAST CANCER SURGERY

Practically all women who have breast cancer go through surgery as part of their treatment, but the type of surgery you are going to have depends on your breast cancer type and stage.

For instance, surgery may be done to:

- Ease symptoms
- know if cancer has spread
- Remove cancer from the body
- Remove the breast(s)
- Reconstruct the breast

Whatever the situation allows, and depending on individual choice, patients may have one of the following types of breast cancer surgery.

Types of breast cancer surgery

Lumpectomy

A lumpectomy is a surgical process that is performed on a breast cancer patient, which is used to remove the cancerous cells and nearby tissues. The reason for this surgical procedure is to remove the cancer tissues while still keeping most of the breast tissues.

Lumpectomy can also be called:

- Breast conservation therapy
- Breast-conserving surgery(BCS)
- Partial mastectomy
- Quadrantectomy
- Segmental mastectomy.

Part of your chest wall may be removed during lumpectomy if the cancer is identified close to this area. Surgeons may likewise decide to remove some of the lymph nodes under your arm if these are concerning regions for cancer.

A lumpectomy is for patients who are diagnosed with breast cancer. It's a good option treatment for patients with early-stage breast cancer. The reason for this surgery is to prevent cancer from spreading to other parts of the body.

Most patients choose to have a lumpectomy because they want to keep their breasts. Patients that choose lumpectomy will still have another treatment, like radiation therapy.

Long-term survival can be the same when compared with mastectomy, if:

- You have little cancer (under 4 cm) in only one breast or tumors that are close together.
- Your surrounding tissues (margins) are clear.

Three elements to think about before deciding on lumpectomy

- Not everybody that has breast cancer is lumpectomy suitable. There are different factors to consider before choosing to do a lumpectomy, like your overall health status, cancer type, and stage. With these factors, you will be able to know if you are a candidate for lumpectomy. You can discuss this with your doctor.

- You need to think about your treatment plan, what are your treatment plans, and how much of your breast tissue you want to get removed. If you want to keep some of your breast tissue, then you have to go for a lumpectomy, although the tumor's size, location, and size of your breast are very important when deciding on your treatment plan.
- You need to think about the importance of keeping your breast tissue.

The side effects of lumpectomy are:

Temporary breast swelling, pain, the scar where your tumor was removed from, swelling in the arm.

Signs of infection at the surgical site after lumpectomy are pain, swelling, fever, fluid discharge, persistent swelling in your arm, and blood collection around the wound site.

Inform your doctor as soon as possible when you see or experience any of these effects and also for follow-up care.

Mastectomy

Mastectomy is recommended for breast cancer patients with an advanced stage of breast cancer or those with a high risk of having breast cancer. During a mastectomy, the entire breast is removed.

Mastectomy may be recommended if you have:

- Ductal carcinoma in situ (DCIS)
- Invasive breast cancer that hasn't spread past the breast
- Paget's disease of the breast
- More than one area of cancer in your breast
- BRCA1 or BRCA2 gene mutation
- Inflammatory breast cancer (IBC)

A mastectomy may be suggested if your cancer recurs after a lumpectomy and radiation.

Men with breast cancer also undergo mastectomy.

Ductal carcinoma in situ (DCIS) and mastectomy

Mastectomy is suggested for DCIS, particularly if:

- Your bosoms are small, and you have a huge area of DCIS.
- DCIS was found in more than one part of your breast ducts.
- Your DCIS is under your nipple.
- Breast conservation therapy will not be able to remove all the DCIS.
- You won't be able to receive radiation therapy.

Types of mastectomies

Total or simple mastectomy: During this surgical procedure, the surgeons remove the whole breast that has cancer. The surgeons may also remove lymph nodes under your arm. Most patients leave the hospital after 24 to 48 hours.

Modified radical mastectomy: During this type of surgery, the surgeons remove the breast, lymph nodes under your arm and the lining over the muscles in your chest.

Skin-sparing mastectomy: During this mastectomy, the surgeon removes the breast tissue, nipple, and areola, leaving the breast skin intact.

Nipple-sparing mastectomy: In this type of mastectomy, the breast tissue is removed, leaving alone the nipple and areola in place.

Double mastectomy: During this type of mastectomy, the two breasts are removed at the same time. This type of mastectomy is for women who are at high risk of getting breast cancer, which includes those with BRCA1 and BRCA2 gene mutations.

Side effects of mastectomy

- Pain near the incision, armpit, and chest wall.
- Blood buildup in the wound area
- A buildup of fluid in the wound area
- Swelling where your breast was removed from
- A buildup of lymph fluid

You should be able to return to some of your normal activities after four weeks.

BREAST RECONSTRUCTION

The choice to go for breast reconstruction after a mastectomy is an individual one. Not all women are advised to have breast reconstructive surgery, and some decide not to seek this type of surgery. Although having this type of surgery that restores the appearance of one or the two breasts helps improve physical, emotional, and social well-being. Discuss the risk of this surgery with your doctors before having it.

Types of breast reconstruction

Immediate breast reconstruction: this type of breast reconstruction is done simultaneously with a mastectomy.

Delayed breast reconstruction: this type of breast reconstruction is done after mastectomy or after treatment ends. This is a better option for those who smoke, have diabetes, and will need radiation therapy after surgery.

Implant-based reconstruction: In this type of reconstruction, the breast is created using silicone gel.

Autologous reconstruction: In this type of breast reconstruction, fat and skin are transplanted from

various parts of the patient body to create another breast.

Final stages of reconstruction

Doctors may recommend these additional techniques for some patients to complete their breast reconstruction process, which are:

- Autologous fat grafting
- Symmetry procedures on the unaffected breast
- Nipple reconstruction
- 3-D nipple tattoo

Conclusion

Cancer is not a death sentence, treatment helps. During your treatment make sure you eat well and take a lot of fruits and vegetables. Also, pray. Wishing you the best in life.

From the author of "Information on breast cancer"

You can do as well get it to have full insight and knowledge about breast cancer.

Thanks for reading.